Introductory Case Studies in Infectious Disease Epidemiology

2nd Edition

Kevin A. Lenhart

Copyright © 2018 Kevin A. Lenhart

All rights reserved.

ISBN: 9781717803368

This set of short case studies is designed to give students an introduction into infectious disease epidemiology. The cases and the case questions have been created to foster discussion about infectious diseases and fundamental epidemiologic principals.

CONTENTS

Case 1 – Hepatitis A

Case 2 - Plague

Case 3 – Dengue Fever

Case 4 - Bacterial Meningitis

Case 5 – Rabies

Case 6 – Shigella

Case 7 – Tuberculosis

Case 8 – Chickenpox

Case Study group Assignment

Individual Practice Assignments

The cases do not depict specific actual events, but rather are a compilation of scenarios that may be observed by epidemiologists in any community on a daily basis.

Public Health is "*...the science and art of preventing disease, prolonging life and promoting health and efficiency through organized community effort for the sanitation of the environment, the control of communicable infections, the education of the individual in personal hygiene, the organization of medical and nursing services for the early diagnosis and preventive treatment of disease, and for the development of the social machinery to insure everyone a standard of living adequate for the maintenance of health, so organizing these benefits as to enable every citizen to realize his birthright of health and longevity.*"

- *C.E.A. Winslow*

Case 1: Hepatitis A

A student from the local community college presents to the on-campus clinic with complaints of fatigue, muscle pain, loss of appetite and a low-grade fever. The student has been feeling ill for the last two days. The Nurse Practitioner notices a yellowing of the student's skin. She orders lab work for the student, including a hepatitis panel.

Over the next three days, four more students present to the clinic with similar symptoms. All five students' lab results show the have Hepatitis A. The local County Health Department is notified and begins an investigation.

All of the students' vaccination and medical records are examined by the Health Department. None have previous Hepatitis A vaccinations. Each student is interviewed and asked question about recent activity, including: roommates, sexual partners, travel history and household members.

The epidemiologist also asks about recent dining locations, drug use and contact with anyone else that may be ill, or show signs of illness.

The Epidemiologist identifies a café on campus as a common dining location for all of the affected students.

The Nurse Practitioner advises the students to stay at home while ill and avoid preparing food for others and sexual activity. She also educates the students on the importance of hand washing.

Since Hepatitis A is a viral infection no medication is recommended in the treatment. Symptoms of the illness, such as nausea and vomiting can be treated.

Case Discussion Question:

1. What are the signs and symptoms of Hepatitis A?

2. Why did the epidemiologist ask about travel history?

3. What are the different ways that the virus can be spread?

4. Why would a restaurant frequented by all of the students be of interest to the Epidemiologist?

5. What preventive measures could the students have taken to avoid contracting Hepatitis A?

6. What are the chances for a full recovery?

Case 2: Plague

Two students participating in an after school agriculture program become suddenly ill. The students present to the local urgent care center with fever, chills and fatigue. Upon examination the physician, Dr. Lloyd, discovers swollen lymph nodes on both students.

Dr. Lloyd takes blood samples from both students, and sends them home to rest.

Within 12 hours the lab has reported that preliminary test indicate the students may have *Yersinia Pestis*, or plague. Dr. Lloyd immediately begins antibiotic treatment for the students and notifies the Health Department.

Within hours of the diagnosis word of the student's illness spreads through the small town, and parents are pulling their kids out of school.

The Health Department begins their investigation and discovers both Students are in Ms. Miller's English class. Both students also are in the afterschool agriculture program and are raising prairie dogs and rabbits for the county fair. It is not believed that the two students have anything else in common, or share any other activities.

36 hours after the samples were sent to the lab Dr. Lloyd receives confirmation that both students are suffering from the plague.

Case Discussion Questions:

1. What are the three types of Yersinia Pestis?

2. Based on the symptoms, what type of plague do the students have?

3. What do you think the likely source of the infection is for these two students?

4. What is the likely mode of transmission? Is that form a transmission common?

5. What is the name for swollen lymph nodes in cases of pestis?

6. Who else may be at risk?

Case 3: Dengue Fever

Three people have tested positive for Dengue fever south of Main Street in Acme County. All three live within a mile of each other and within 400 yards of a low-lying swamp area near a middle school. This area has never had a reported case of Dengue fever.

All three patients presented to the doctor with similar symptoms of fever, nausea and vomiting. The cases began showing symptoms within a one week period. The cases range in age from 27 to 66. Two cases have no recent travel history, and one has history of recent travel to an area that has no known dengue activity. The only common factor shared by the cases is geographic location.

Parents are calling asking for the Health Department to cancel all outdoor school activities. Mosquito control is being asked to spray the entire county, but only has the resources to spray about one third of the county.

The County mayor has asked the Health department to advise on prevention methods and to educate the community on risk factors.

Case Discussion Questions:

1) What is the mode of transmission of Dengue fever?

2) What is the treatment for dengue fever?

3) What is the incubation period for Dengue fever?

4) What prevention activates should the Health Department recommend?

5) Who is at risk in this community for contracting the Dengue fever?

6) What are the chances for recovery for the three with Dengue?

7) Are their surveillance methods that are used in other communities that may be adopted by Acme County in the future?

Case 4: Bacterial Meningitis

A student at the local High School was admitted to the hospital on Monday with sudden onset of headache, fever, nausea and sensitivity to light. The patient also presented with a stiff neck. A spinal tap (lumbar puncture) was performed, and sent to the lab. Results indicate that the student was positive for nesseria meningitis.

Rumors about the infection have spread around the school. Parents are concerned for their children's safety. The Health Department and the school have become overwhelmed with calls.

The Health Department has begun investigating known contacts of the case.

The student is a member of the school soccer team and is active in afterschool activities. The list of known contacts has grown to over 70. The investigation has expended to neighboring communities when the school soccer teams has traveled for games.

The local Health Department has asked for assistance from the CDC Epidemic Intelligence Service (EIS) since the case contact investigation has grown larger than the small community can handle.

Case Discussion Questions:

1) What is the mode of transmission of Nessseria Meningitidis?

2) What is the treatment?

3) Who is at risk of exposure?

4) What is treatment for potential exposure?

5) What are the chances for recovery?

6) Are there potential prevention measure that should be put into place?

7) How should the Health Department proceed with the investigation?

Case 5: Rabies

A fifty year old man reported to Animal Control that his two dogs were attacked by a raccoon earlier in the day. Because the attack occurred during the day, Animal Control is concerned the raccoon may be rabid. They have verified both dogs have current rabies vaccinations. Animal Control has notified the Health Department of the attack, and they have begun an investigation.

While the man was not bitten or scratched by the raccoon, he did attend to the dogs' wounds. The Health Department has recommended that he receive post exposure treatment.

Over the past three months there have been reports of two other raccoons attacking pets in the same community. In all instances the pets have had current vaccinations, and the raccoons have not been killed or captured.

Animal Control has begun patrolling the area daily. They are picking up all stray animals within a two mile radius of the attack. The Health Department has sent out media advisories warning residents of the potential dangers rabies exposure and the importance of keeping pets vaccinated.

Case Questions:

1) What is the mode of transmission of Rabies?

2) What is the treatment?

3) What is treatment for potential exposure?

4) What are the chances for recovery?

5) Other than vaccination, are there potential prevention measure that should be put into place?

6) How should the Health Department proceed with the investigation?

7) Can the local government do anything to help prevent the spread of rabies?

Case 6: Shigella

Sunday afternoon 320 people attended a church picnic. The church provided hamburgers and hot dogs. Everyone else brought side items that they shared with other attendees. The picnic was held outside in a park next to the church. The temperature reached ninety degrees Fahrenheit.

The following day, Pastor Kelley stayed home sick from work. He had developed a fever and stomach cramps. He received a call later in the day that several other members of the church had developed similar symptoms, some who were also suffering from diarrhea.

The next morning Pastor Kelley visited his physician, Dr. Hubley, since his symptoms had not improved. He mentioned that several other members of the church, who all had attended the picnic were ill as well. Dr. Hubley collected a stool sample and notified the health Department that there was a possible foodborne illness outbreak in the community.

The Health Department began investigating and found nineteen people who reported becoming ill within two days of attending the church picnic.

Lab results returned to Dr. Hubley showed that Pastor Kelley was positive for *Shigella Sonnei*. Since his symptoms were beginning to subside, no antibiotics were prescribed.

Several others who became ill were treated and are expected to make a full recovery.

Case Discussion Questions:

1) What steps should the Health Department take next to try and determine the specific source of the outbreak?

1) Did Dr. Hubley do the right thing reporting her suspicion of an outbreak to the Health department?

2) Would this be considered an outbreak?

3) What could the Church have done to ensure proper food handling at a picnic?

4) What are the chances for full recovery for the nineteen people who became ill?

5) What is the typical incubation period for shigella?

Case 7: Tuberculosis

During a routine history and physical of an inmate at the county jail, it was noticed that he had experienced weight loss of eighteen pounds since his initial incarceration eight months earlier. He also had developed a cough and reported having a slight fever and night sweats for the last two weeks. A routine TB shin test was planted and the inmate was placed on the cold treatment protocol.

The inmate is a 51 year old male who self-reports as homeless. He has no immediate family and has been incarcerated in the jail for eight months.

Results from the TB Skin test were positive, and a chest x-ray was scheduled for the following day. The inmate was placed in airborne isolation and staff was notified to take precautions until the results of further testing returned.

The chest x-ray showed a lesion in the inmate's lung in the lower right lobe. The Health Department was notified and their infectious disease expert reviewed the clinical notes and diagnostics. An Acid-fast Bacilli (ASB) test was ordered and the jail was given instructions on proper collection of the sputum samples.

The initial results from the sputum showed a positive stain for AFB. The Health Department was notified and the inmate was started on treatment.

The Health Department had already begun to investigate possible contacts. As that continued, it became obvious that in such close quarters as a correctional facility, this inmate had come into close contact with many staff and other inmates.

Case Discussion Questions:

1) What would be the next step for the Health Department after identifying contacts?

2) Are there factors that would make inmates in a correctional facility more susceptible, or at higher risk for contracting TB?

3) What are some of the airborne precautions the jail should implement when they suspect someone may have TB?

4) How long after treatment should the inmate be kept in isolation?

5) Did the inmate have active TB? If so, how would that differ from latent TB?

Case 8: Chickenpox

While working the night shift of the urgent care clinic, Dr. Patton has a six-year-old male patient present with complaints of fever, headache and tiredness. His mother states that the symptoms started one day before.

Upon examination, Dr. Patton identifies a rash with small raised bumps on the child's chest and torso.

The child's mother states that the child did not complete his recommended vaccinations for childhood illness. She states that she felt that there were too many vaccinations with possible complications and it would be detrimental to the child's health to complete the recommended vaccinations. She also tells Dr. Patton two other children in the household are unvaccinated and have been in recent contact with the patient. Dr. Patton stated that he believes that, while uncommon, the child is suffering from chickenpox and the other children have likely been exposed as well.

Dr. Patton also explained that any adults who did not have previous history of chickenpox and had not been vaccinated were at potential risk of developing the infection

.

Case Discussion Questions:

1) How long is the patient contagious?

2) Who else was potentially exposed to the child while he was infectious?

3) what are the potential complications from chickenpox infection?

4) what other diseases without child with current vaccinations be susceptible to?

Case Study Group Assignment

1) Groups are to present their case study as if they were the epidemiologists, demonstrating a knowledge of the principals and procedures of epidemiology.
    a. Outline the investigation process.
    b. Address community concerns and potential community concerns.

2) Develop a press release and educational materials related to your case.

3) Create a video public service announcement (PSA) related to your related case.

Individual Practice Assignment

Assignment 1:
Visit the Centers for Disease Control and Prevention website (https://www.cdc.gov/) Research an infectious disease not included in the current case studies. Using the chain of infection, identify each link in the chain, and how it is related to the disease you've researched.

Individual Practice Assignment

Assignment 2:

Visit the World Health Organization website (http://www.who.int/en/) and identify a current outbreak in another part of the world currently being investigated by the WHO. Identify the agent and mode of transmission.

Individual Practice Assignment

Assignment 3:

Visit the American Public Health Association (APHA) website (https://www.apha.org/) Visit the Career Development section of the page. Identify three different jobs in the epidemiology field.

Individual Practice Assignment

Assignment 4:
Visit the CDC website for emerging infectious diseases (https://wwwnc.cdc.gov/eid) and identify current ongoing research in infectious disease. What are the current priorities for the CDC in infectious disease research?

www.ingramcontent.com/pod-product-compliance
Lightning Source LLC
Chambersburg PA
CBHW031508210526
45463CB00003B/1137